Mucusless Diet Healing System
For Beginners

Revitalize Your Life By Embracing the
Mucusless Diet for Holistic Healing.

Title:
Mucusless Diet Healing System
For Beginners

Subtitle

Revitalize Your Life By Embracing the Mucusless Diet for Holistic Healing.

Copyright © 2023 by (Guillermo Bode MD)

Printed in the United States of America.

ISBN: 9798872613008

TABLE OF CONTENT

INTRODUCTION

In the maze of dietary paradigms and wellness philosophies, there is one particular approach that has endured the test of time and continued to captivate the attention of individuals who are looking for not just a diet but also an all-encompassing healing system. This approach is known as the Mucusless Diet. The purpose of this introduction is to shed light on a transforming path toward health and vitality by delving into the beginnings, background, and visionary figure behind the Mucusless Diet Healing System.

Background and Origin of the Mucusless Diet

The early 20th century saw a rise in interest in complementary medicine and holistic approaches to well-being, which is when the Mucusless Diet first emerged. As the name implies, the goal of the Mucusless Diet is to prevent and improve health by removing foods that cause mucus from one's diet.

This diet plan is based on the idea that some foods, especially those made from processed foods and animal products, cause the body to produce too much mucus. It is hypothesized that this extra mucus serves as a haven for infections, toxins, and other dangerous chemicals, which can cause a variety of health problems, from chronic diseases to digestive disturbances.

The German naturopath and health educator Arnold Ehret, the creator of the Mucusless Diet, was instrumental in spreading awareness of this ground-breaking nutritional strategy. Ehret, who was born in 1866, underwent a journey of self-discovery and became passionate about natural medicine as a result of his health issues. He was suffering from several illnesses, including asthma, and was unable to find any relief from them using traditional medicine. His health didn't start to improve until he started using alternative treatment techniques, namely fasting and a plant-based diet.

Arnold Ehret's groundbreaking book, "The Mucusless Diet Healing System," which was initially released in 1922, was the result of his observations and experiences. This groundbreaking book described the tenets and protocols of the Mucusless Diet, offering a comprehensive approach that covered fasting, detoxification, and lifestyle choices in addition to nutritional recommendations. As word of Ehret's teachings spread, people looking for holistic approaches to health and wellness began to take notice.

The Visionary Behind the Mucusless Diet Healing System

It becomes clear that Arnold Ehret was a visionary whose contributions to natural health and wellness have had a lasting influence. His worldview encompassed a comprehensive approach to health that integrated mental, physical, and spiritual well-being, going beyond food advice.

By stressing the body's capacity to cure itself through appropriate diet and lifestyle choices, Ehret questioned the then-dominant medical paradigm. His support of a diet rich in fresh produce, fruits, and non-mucus-forming foods was in line with naturopathy's core beliefs and paved the way for a new wave of health enthusiasts and professionals.

Ehret's teachings revolved around the idea of interior purity, which is attained by avoiding foods that cause mucus and letting the body go through a detoxification process. His conviction that the body has the innate capacity to repair and cure itself struck a chord with people looking for non-invasive medical methods and pharmaceutical interventions as alternatives.

Arnold Ehret's influence on the Mucusless Diet Healing System extends beyond his written writings and may be seen in the groups and societies that have adopted his ideas. Through study groups, fasting retreats, and online forums, the Mucusless Diet has attracted a devoted fan base that keeps investigating and putting Ehret's ideas into practice in the quest for vibrant health.

Recognizing the Mucusless Diet as more than just a collection of dietary recommendations is crucial in appreciating Ehret's visionary role since it signifies a paradigm shift in the way we view and approach health. Ehret's influence is still felt in the broader framework of natural health and holistic living, as well as in the ongoing observance of his dietary guidelines.

CHAPTER 1: UNDERSTANDING THE MUCUSLESS DIET

In the pursuit of optimal health and well-being, the choices that one makes about one's nutrition are of equal importance. The Mucusless Diet, which is founded on ideas that go beyond simple dietary requirements, provides a fresh viewpoint on the connection that exists between food, the body, and the process of healing. The purpose of this investigation is to provide a comprehensive understanding of the Mucusless Diet by elucidating its definition, the fundamental principles that underlie it, the physiological function of mucus, the healing mechanisms that it supports, and the essential components that make up this revolutionary dietary system.

Definition and Principles of the Mucusless Diet

At its core, the Mucusless Diet is a nutritional philosophy that is predicated on the concept that some foods contribute to the creation of excess mucus in the body, which in turn leads to a variety of health problems. It is the major objective of the diet to avoid or reduce the consumption of foods that produce mucus and to cultivate a cleaner interior environment that is conducive to increased health and vigor.

The following are the fundamental ideas of the Mucusless Diet:

- Plant-Based Emphasis: The diet promotes a primarily plant-based diet with a focus on seasonal produce. These foods are thought to assist the body's natural healing processes and are classified as non-mucus-forming foods.

- Foods that Form Mucus: Foods that form mucus, like meat, dairy, refined grains, and processed foods, are either avoided or severely limited. The reasoning for this is that these foods cause the body to produce more mucus, which is thought to serve as a haven for germs and poisons.

- Comprehending Food Combining: The goal of proper food combining is to improve the absorption of nutrients and digestion. The Mucusless Diet offers precise recommendations for blending various food kinds to enhance the digestive system's performance.

- Intermittent Fasting: The Mucusless Diet incorporates fasting as a healing and detoxifying therapy. It is thought that fasting periods enable the body to refocus energy on detoxification and regrowth.

- Hydration: To assist the body's detoxification activities and preserve general health, an adequate intake of water is advised. It is believed that maintaining optimal physiological function and eliminating toxins require adequate hydration.

The Role of Mucus in the Body

Gaining an understanding of mucus's function in the body is essential to understanding the Mucusless Diet's tenets. The body uses mucus, a slippery, viscous substance made by mucous membranes, for several vital processes. It functions as a barrier of defense, lubricating and moistening surfaces, including those in the digestive and respiratory systems.

Mucus is essential for capturing and removing infections, irritants, and foreign particles in a healthy state. Nonetheless, proponents of the Mucusless Diet contend that difficulties may result from producing too much mucus. From this angle, it is thought that some foods cause the overproduction of mucus, which in turn

13

fosters the growth of pathogenic microbes and the retention of poisons.

People who follow the Mucusless Diet try to eat less of the foods that are believed to be associated with excessive mucus formation. This decrease is therefore thought to lessen the load on the body's defense systems naturally and encourage a healthier interior environment.

How the Mucusless Diet Supports Healing

The Mucusless Diet is not only a collection of food restrictions; rather, it is an all-encompassing therapeutic strategy that targets the underlying causes of a wide variety of health problems. Several different mechanisms are responsible for the therapeutic effects of the Mucus-Free Diet, including the following:

- Detoxification: One way to help with detoxification is to cut back or eliminate meals that make mucus. Reducing the amount of things that are supposed to cause mucus buildup helps the body go through a purging process, releasing waste and toxins that have been accumulated.

- Enhanced Digestion: The digestive process is optimized by placing a focus on plant-based, non-mucus-forming diets and properly combining nutrients. Better nutrient absorption and utilization can boost general health through improved digestion.

- Decreased Inflammation: The Mucusless Diet's proponents argue that cutting out specific inflammatory foods helps lower the body's overall level of inflammation. Reducing chronic inflammation is thought to be essential to the healing process because it is associated with several illnesses.

- Microbiome balancing: It is thought that the plant-based diet, in conjunction with periodic fasting, has a beneficial effect on the gut microbiome. Enhanced immune response and general health are linked to a balanced and diversified microbiome.

- Nutrient Density: Foods that do not create mucus, such as fruits and vegetables, are high in fiber, antioxidants, and vital nutrients. The goal of the mucusless diet is to give the body the components it needs for maximum healing and function.

Key Components of a Mucusless Diet

To put the Mucusless Diet into practice, one must make a deliberate choice of foods that are by its guiding principles or principles. Although tastes and tolerances can vary from person to person, the following are widely considered to be essential components of a mucus-free diet:

- Fruits: An essential component of the Mucusless Diet is fresh, ripe fruit. These consist of a wide range of fruits, including melons, grapes, citrus fruits, apples, and berries. Eating fruits in their whole, unadulterated form is the focus.

- Vegetables: A wide variety of cooked and raw veggies are recommended. A variety of nutrients can be found in leafy greens, cruciferous veggies, root vegetables, and other vibrant vegetables.

- Non-Mucus-Forming Grains: When consumed in moderation, whole grains like quinoa, brown rice, and oats are deemed appropriate. It is thought that these grains are less likely to develop mucus than refined grains.

- Nuts and Seeds: Due to their high nutritional value, raw, unsalted nuts and seeds are part of the Mucusless Diet. Nuts and seeds that fit the diet's tenets include almonds, flaxseeds, and sunflower seeds.

- Herbs and Spices: To add taste to food without introducing substances that cause mucus formation, fresh herbs and spices like turmeric, parsley, ginger, and cilantro are utilized.

- Water: An essential component of the Mucusless Diet is hydration. The best beverage to aid the body's natural detoxification processes is pure water.

Individual customization is encouraged based on criteria such as personal health objectives, dietary preferences, and any current health issues. Although the Mucusless Diet provides a fundamental framework, it is important to note that it is open to adaptation. When approaching the diet, it is vital to do so with mindfulness and an understanding of the specific requirements of the individual.

CHAPTER 2: TRANSITIONING TO A MUCUSLESS DIET

Deciding to embark on a path towards a mucusless diet is a considerable transformation in both one's lifestyle and one's dietary habits. This transformation is not simply a change in the foods that you consume; rather, it is an approach to health that takes a comprehensive perspective. During this investigation, we will walk you through the fundamental aspects of making the switch to a mucus-free diet. These aspects include evaluating your current eating habits, deciding whether to make the switch gradually or immediately, developing strategies to overcome obstacles and detox symptoms, and developing a Mucus-free Diet plan that is both balanced and sustainable.

Assessing Your Current Dietary Habits

You must take an objective look at your present eating habits before beginning the Mucusless Diet. Think about the kinds of foods you usually eat, how you eat, and the extent to which these choices follow the guidelines of the Mucusless Diet.

- Food Journaling: Keep track of everything you eat and drink for a week in a food journal. This diary will be an invaluable resource for spotting trends, identifying foods that cause mucus formation, and comprehending your dietary choices.

- Analyze the nutrients in your current diet by conducting a nutrient analysis. Observe how your diet distributes the macronutrients (proteins, fats, and carbohydrates) and micronutrients (vitamins and minerals). You can use this analysis to pinpoint places that could require modifications.

- Recognizing Mucus-Forming Foods: Get acquainted with typical meals that cause mucus, including meat, dairy, processed foods, and refined grains. Making educated decisions during the shift will be made easier if you can identify these foods in your existing diet.

Gradual vs. Immediate Transition

The choice to switch to a mucusless diet gradually or all at once is a personal one that is impacted by a variety of factors, including preparedness for change, personal preferences, and health concerns.

Gradual Shift: A gradual transition turns out to be a more sustainable strategy for a lot of people. The body can adjust to dietary changes more easily when mucus-forming foods are gradually reduced while non-mucus-forming food consumption is increased. Additionally, by using this method, detoxification symptoms can be reduced.

Immediate Transition: Some folks could decide to start a mucusless diet right away. This bold move necessitates a bigger change in a shorter amount of time. Although it can result in quicker detoxification and possibly quicker health improvements, it can also present difficulties, particularly for people used to a very different diet.

Whichever strategy you decide on, it's critical to pay attention to how your body feels and how it reacts to nutritional adjustments. If you want to make a gradual change, you may establish specific goals, such as cutting back on meat or dairy over a few weeks. If you want to make an immediate transfer, you would have to switch to non-mucus-forming items completely.

Overcoming Challenges and Detox Symptoms

Shifting to a Mucusless Diet may cause difficulties and symptoms of detoxification until the body gets used to the new eating pattern. A seamless and long-lasting transfer depends on recognizing and resolving these issues.

- **Common Challenges:**

Cravings: During the shift, it's normal to experience cravings for familiar meals, particularly ones that are heavy in sugar, salt, or fat. Use a range of flavors in your meals to stave off cravings, and cut back on processed foods gradually.

Social Pressures: If your new food choices deviate from the norm, social situations and peer pressure may provide difficulties. Tell your loved ones about your nutritional choices, and ask for their assistance as you pursue wellness.

Detox Symptoms:

Fatigue: One of the most typical detox symptoms is feeling exhausted or having little energy. Make sure you are getting enough sleep, drink enough water, and think about including foods high in energy, including fruits and leafy greens, in your diet.

Headaches: Sometimes headaches are brought on by detoxification. To relieve symptoms, drink plenty of water, get enough rest, and think about including foods or herbal teas high in magnesium.

Digestive Changes: During detox, it's normal to see changes in bowel movements. Consuming more fruits and vegetables to increase fiber intake can promote a healthy digestive system.

Creating a Balanced and Sustainable Mucusless Diet Plan

For long-term success, a well-balanced and long-lasting Mucusless Diet plan must be created. The following important factors should help you create a plan that complements your tastes and goals:

- Variety of Fruits and Vegetables: To guarantee a wide range of nutrients, emphasize a variety of fruits and vegetables. To optimize the nutritional advantages, incorporate a variety of colors, textures, and flavors.

- Protein Sources: A Mucusless Diet minimizes animal products, but it's still necessary to make sure you're getting enough protein

31

from plants. To satisfy your protein needs, include whole grains, legumes, nuts, and seeds.

- Healthy Fats: To support vital body functions, include foods high in healthy fats, such as avocados, nuts, and seeds. These fats support general health and provide you with energy.

- Hydration: Make staying hydrated a top priority by drinking lots of clean water all day long. Infused water and herbal teas can spice up your daily hydration regimen.

- Food Combining Ideas: To improve digestion, become familiar with these principles. Carefully matching meals can improve the absorption of nutrients and reduce gastrointestinal distress.

- Meal Planning: To guarantee a varied and well-balanced diet, plan your meals. Try different flavors, recipes, and cooking techniques to add interest and enjoyment to your meals.

- Listen to Your Body: Observe the reactions that various foods have on your body. Modify your diet if you feel uncomfortable or observe any particular symptoms. Since the Mucusless Diet is flexible, individual differences are to be expected.

CHAPTER 3: MUCUSLESS DIET FOODS AND RECIPES

When you start a mucus-free diet, you open up a whole new world of vivid, nutrient-dense foods that facilitate the natural healing processes that occur within your body. This section delves into the fundamental aspects of the Mucusless Diet, including an examination of the differences between alkaline and acidic foods, an emphasis on the fruits and vegetables that are recommended, a discussion of the role that grains, nuts, and seeds play, the provision of sample recipes for the Mucusless Diet, and the provision of seven sample meal plans to assist you on your journey toward physical and mental health through the realm of food.

Alkaline vs. Acidic Foods

It is suggested that alkaline-forming foods contribute to a cleaner internal environment, which is supported by the Mucusless Diet, which lays a considerable emphasis on the alkaline-ash-forming characteristic of specifically selected meals. To make educated decisions about one's diet, it is necessary to have a solid understanding of the alkaline and acidic classifications of foods.

- **Alkaline-Forming Foods:**

Fruits: The majority of fruits, especially those with a high water content like melons, berries, and citrus fruits, are thought to generate an alkaline environment.

Veggies: An essential part of the Mucusless Diet, leafy greens, cruciferous vegetables, and root vegetables are alkaline-forming.

Herbs and Spices: A variety of alkaline-forming herbs and spices, including parsley, ginger, and cilantro, can be used to add taste to food.

- **Acidic-Forming Foods:**

Animal Products: In the Mucusless Diet, meat, dairy, and eggs are typically categorized as items that generate acidity.

Processed Foods: Sugary snacks, refined cereals, and processed foods frequently produce acids.

Some Grains: Although entire grains are generally thought to be neutral or slightly alkaline, some Mucusless Diet proponents advise restricting or eliminating specific grains that might be thought to be acidic.

It's crucial to remember that the alkaline-ash-forming theory is only a basic classification system for foods. A food's total effect on the pH of the body depends on several variables, such as the individual's metabolism and the diet's general composition.

Recommended Fruits and Vegetables

The Mucusless Diet places a strong emphasis on fruits and vegetables, which are great sources of a wide variety of nutrients, including vitamins, minerals, fiber, and antioxidants. Some options that are advised are as follows:

- **Fruits:**

Berries: Antioxidant-rich berries including blueberries, strawberries, raspberries, and blackberries can be incorporated into the Mucusless Diet.

Citrus Fruits: Vitamin C and reviving flavors are contributed by oranges, grapefruits, lemons, and limes.

Melons: Honeydew, cantaloupe, and watermelon are alkalizing and hydrating options.

Apples: A fruit with many uses, they can be eaten on their own or added to a variety of meals.

• **Vegetables:**

Leafy Greens: A great source of vitamins and minerals are spinach, kale, Swiss chard, and collard greens.

Cruciferous Vegetables: There are several health advantages to eating cabbage, Brussels sprouts, cauliflower, and broccoli.

Root Vegetables: Beets, carrots, and sweet potatoes give meals sweetness and nutrition.

You can consume these fruits and vegetables raw, juiced, or combined with other ingredients to make salads, smoothies, and other dishes.

Grains, Nuts, and Seeds in the Mucusless Diet

Even though the Mucusless Diet places a considerable amount of focus on fresh fruits and vegetables, there is still room for specific grains, nuts, and seeds that are by the principles of the diet.

- **Grains:**

Quinoa: A complete protein source that is adaptable and high in nutrients.

Brown rice is a whole grain that is high in fiber and vital elements.

Oats: A heart-healthy grain that tastes good in oatmeal and overnight oats, among other variations.

- **Nuts and Seeds:**

Almonds: Packed with protein, vitamin E, and good fats.

Chia seeds: Rich in fiber, antioxidants, and omega-3 fatty acids.

Omega-3s and lignans, which may have positive effects on health, can be found in flaxseeds.

You may add extra nutrition, texture, and flavor to Mucusless Diet meals by including these grains, nuts, and seeds.

Sample Mucusless Diet Recipes

To fully realize the culinary potential of the Mucus-Free Diet, it is necessary to experiment with food recipes that are both delicious and healthful. Here are three sample recipes to get you started on your adventure through the world of mucus-free cuisine:

1. Mucusless Green Smoothie:

Ingredients:

- One cup of de-stemmed kale leaves
- half a cucumber, sliced and peeled
- one cored and sliced green apple and one squeezed lemon
- One spoonful of chia seeds
- one cup of coconut water or water
- Cubes of ice (optional)

Instructions:

- All of the components should be placed in a blender.

- Puree till it is silky smooth and creamy.

- If additional water is required to get the desired consistency, add it.

- After pouring it into a glass, you can consume it with ice cubes if you so wish.

2. Quinoa and Vegetable Stir-Fry:

Ingredients:

- 1 cup of quinoa, cooked.

- broccoli florets in a cup.

- One bell pepper cut thinly.

- One julienned carrot.

- Add 1/2 cup of trimmed snap peas.

- two minced garlic cloves.

- One tablespoon of soy sauce or tamari.

- One tablespoon of sesame oil.

- One tablespoon of extra virgin olive oil.

- As a garnish, add sesame seeds.

Instructions:

- In a large saucepan, bring the olive oil to a temperature of medium.

- Sauté the garlic until it achieves a fragrant state.
- Make sure to include snap peas, carrots, bell peppers, and broccoli in the pan.
- The vegetables should be stir-fried until they are crisp-tender.
- Incorporate quinoa that has been cooked, tamari or soy sauce, and sesame oil. To combine, give it a toss.
- Continue to cook for an additional two to three minutes, or until everything is completely hot.
- Before serving, sprinkle the dish with sesame seeds.

3. Citrus and Berry Salad:

Ingredients:

- Two cups of mixed berries (strawberries, blueberries, raspberries).
- Peel and segment one orange.
- Peel, cut, and slice one kiwi.
- 1 tablespoon finely chopped fresh mint.
- One spoonful of maple syrup or honey (optional).

Instructions:

- Put the kiwi slices, orange segments, and mixed berries into a big bowl and mix them.
- Sprinkle the fruit with mint that has been chopped.

- If you want to add more sweetness, you can drizzle honey or maple syrup over the dish.
- To incorporate the ingredients, give the salad a light toss.
- Before serving, let the dish stay in the refrigerator for half an hour.

Sample Meal Plans

Developing meal plans that are both well-balanced and varied is necessary to maintain a mucusless diet. With the following seven sample meal plans, you will be able to navigate through a week of eating without mucus:

Day 1:

- Mucusless Green Smoothie for breakfast.
- Quinoa and vegetable stir-fry for lunch.
- Steamed broccoli and baked sweet potatoes for dinner.

Day 2:

- Berry and Citrus Salad for breakfast.
- Lunch would be vegetable and lentil soup.

- Dinner is roasted asparagus paired with grilled portobello mushrooms.

Day 3:

- Breakfast consists of Chia seeds and overnight oats with almond milk.
- Lunch is a mixed greens and chickpea salad.
- Dinner is stir-fried tofu and vegetables served in a brown rice bowl.

Day 4:

- Fruit salad with mint for breakfast.
- Quinoa salad with avocado, tomato, and cucumber for lunch.
- Dinner is cherry tomatoes and pesto-topped zucchini noodles.

Day 5:

Chia seed pudding and fresh berries for breakfast.

Lunch consists of corn and black bean-stuffed bell peppers.

Dinner is Brussels sprouts and roasted cauliflower with herbs.

Day 6:

- Smoothie with almond butter and apples for breakfast.
- Lunch is a salad of spinach, mushrooms, and balsamic vinaigrette.
- Dinner is stuffed with acorn squash vegetables and lentils.

Day 7:

Toast with avocado on whole grain bread for breakfast.

Lunch is Kale and Cabbage Slaw with Dressing of Tahini.

Dinner is baked eggplant flavored with basil and tomato.

These sample meal plans demonstrate the versatility and adaptability of the Mucusless Diet by providing a wide range of flavors, textures, and nutrients to choose from. Feel free to modify them according to your preferences, dietary requirements, and the amount of food you want to consume.

CHAPTER 4: DETOXIFICATION AND HEALING

The Mucusless Diet is not an exception to the rule that the concept of detoxification occupies a prominent place among individuals who are striving to achieve optimal health. This section delves into the complexities of the detoxification process, investigates the various detoxification techniques that are commonly used, elucidates the connection between the Mucusless Diet and healing, and presents testimonials and success stories that are evidence of the transformative power of this holistic approach.

Understanding the Detoxification Process

The elimination of waste products and toxins is the goal of detoxification, which is a natural process that occurs continuously throughout the body. To keep the body in a condition of internal equilibrium requires several different organs and systems to collaborate. The liver, kidneys, lungs, skin, and digestive system are the key organs that are involved in the detoxification process.

- Liver: The liver is an essential organ for detoxification because it breaks down and neutralizes toxins into substances that are soluble in water and may be excreted in the urine or bile.

- Kidneys: These organs produce urine to eliminate poisons by filtering waste materials from circulation. Sufficient hydration aids in the kidneys' removal of pollutants.

- Lungs: The lungs aid in the removal of pollutants by expelling carbon dioxide and other volatile compounds during respiration.

- Skin: Sweating is one way the skin helps the body get rid of pollutants. Sweating-inducing activities, including working out or sauna trips, help the skin perform its detoxifying function.

- Digestive System: Waste is removed by the digestive system through bowel motions. Toxin elimination is facilitated by a healthy digestive tract, which also enhances general well-being.

- The Mucusless Diet is sometimes viewed as assisting the body's natural detoxification processes because of its emphasis on meals that don't generate mucus and the elimination of potentially hazardous items. The Mucusless Diet's proponents contend that by consuming fewer items that cause mucus, the body's detoxifying organs are freely taxed and may work at their best.

Common Detoxification Techniques

Even though the Mucus-Free Diet is inherently structured to assist the body in its detoxification processes, there are extra approaches that can complement and enhance the detoxification journey:

Hydration: Drinking enough water is essential for maintaining kidney function and eliminating toxins through the urine. Herbal teas are also acceptable, particularly those that are renowned for their ability to cleanse.

Intermittent Fasting: It is thought that short- or long-term fasts provide a respite for the digestive system, enabling the body to focus its energy on the processes of cleansing and repair.

Exercise: Moving about encourages sweating, circulation, and lymphatic drainage, all of which help the body get rid of pollutants. Pick enjoyable hobbies, including yoga, weight training, jogging, or strolling.

Sauna & Steam Therapy: Sweating with heat promotes the skin's natural elimination of toxins. Sauna treatments can assist the body's natural detoxification processes soothingly and efficiently.

Deep Breathing: Exercises involving deep breathing improve the body's oxygenation, which supports lung health and cellular detoxification.

Colon Cleansing: To support colon health and improve waste evacuation, some people use techniques such as enemas or colon hydrotherapy.

It's crucial to proceed cautiously with detoxification and select techniques that suit your particular requirements and state of health. It is best to speak with a healthcare provider before beginning any rigorous detoxification procedures.

The Connection Between Mucusless Diet and Healing

The Mucusless Diet, which emphasizes the avoidance of foods that generate mucus and are thought to play a role in the onset of disease, is inextricably related to the healing process. The following fundamental ideas can be used to examine the relationship between the Mucusless Diet and healing:

- Interior Cleanliness: The idea of internal cleanliness is essential to the Mucusless Diet. The diet attempts to establish an interior environment that is less conducive to the multiplication of toxins, infections, and hazardous substances by lowering the intake of foods that cause mucus.

- Nutrient Density: Eating a lot of fruits and vegetables, in particular, is encouraged by the Mucusless Diet. These foods enhance the body's general health and vigor by providing crucial vitamins, minerals, antioxidants, and fiber.

- Decreased Inflammation: Many chronic diseases have an inflammatory component. The Mucusless Diet may help to lessen inflammation in the body by limiting inflammatory foods, creating a healing environment.

- Improved Digestion: Proper food combination and the addition of foods that are readily digested can result in better digestion and absorption of nutrients.

Effective digestion facilitates the body's capacity to absorb vital nutrients for restoration.

- Comprehensive Approach: The Mucusless Diet promotes a holistic approach to well-being that goes beyond dietary decisions. A healthy diet, regular exercise, stress reduction, and enough sleep are all essential to the healing process.

Anecdotal accounts and testimonies from people who have followed the Mucusless Diet suggest a variety of health benefits, including increased energy, improved digestion, and relief from various health concerns, despite the paucity of scientific data supporting these principles.

Testimonials and Success Stories

Testimonials and success stories offer personal narratives of people who have adopted the Mucusless Diet and found favorable results. These personal accounts provide insights into the possible effects of the diet on individual health and well-being, although they are subjective and cannot apply to everyone.

- Better Digestive Health: A lot of testimonies point to better digestive health, including relief from constipation, gas, and bloating. Proponents credit these advantages to the removal of foods that cause mucus formation and the encouragement of an environment that is more alkaline within.

- Weight control: A few people claim that the Mucusless Diet helps them successfully control their weight and even lose weight. These results might be attributed to the reduction of processed foods and the concentration of nutrient-dense, low-calorie diets.

- Enhanced Vitality and Energy: Testimonials frequently speak of an increase in general vitality and energy levels. Proponents of the Mucusless Diet explain these modifications as the body's capacity to divert digestive energy to processes of detoxification and repair.

- Resolving Particular Health Problems: Some people talk about how they were able to alleviate or resolve particular health problems, like allergies, skin diseases, and respiratory ailments. Though everyone's experience is different, some people feel that the Mucusless Diet was a big part of their recovery.

It's crucial to view testimonies critically and recognize that every person's health experience is unique. Adopting the Mucusless Diet may yield tremendous benefits for many individuals, but it may not have the same effect on others. It is essential to get advice from medical experts and take into account unique health circumstances.

CHAPTER 5: BENEFITS OF THE MUCUSLESS DIET

The Mucusless Diet, which is based on the principle of avoiding foods that produce mucus, has garnered interest because it can promote holistic well-being to its followers. Managing weight, improving mental clarity and emotional well-being, and improving digestion and elimination are just some of the many benefits that are discussed in this section of the article. Other benefits include increased energy and vitality, improved digestion and elimination, and improved energy and vitality.

Improved Digestion and Elimination

Internal Harmony Through Dietary Choices

One of the main advantages of the Mucusless Diet is that it improves excretion and digestion. The diet's main goal is to foster the right meal combinations and non-mucus-forming foods to optimize the digestive system from the inside out.

Minimizing Digestive Discomfort: Cutting back on or giving up foods that make mucus, like dairy and processed meals, may help reduce discomfort in the digestive tract. Following the Mucusless Diet, many people report feeling free bloated, gassy, and indigestion.

Encouraging Frequent Removal: It is thought that focusing on fruits and vegetables high in fiber and avoiding items that cause constipation can help maintain regular bowel movements. A diet high in plant-based meals and adequate fluids helps to keep the digestive system in good condition.

Optimizing Nutrient Absorption: Eating meals high in nutrients is encouraged by the Mucusless Diet, which may improve the absorption of important vitamins and minerals. It is believed that following appropriate food combination guidelines may improve nutritional absorption and digestion.

Anecdotal comments from those who have followed the Mucusless Diet frequently highlight improvements in digestive health, despite the paucity of scientific studies particularly addressing the benefits of this dietary strategy for the digestive system.

Increased Energy and Vitality

Revitalizing the Body and Mind

Having more energy and general vitality is another well-reported advantage of the mucusless diet. Dietary advocates speculate that this increase in energy is a result of removing foods that cause mucus and placing more of an emphasis on nutrient-dense plant-based diets.

Redirected Energy: It is thought that cutting back on heavy, mucus-forming foods releases energy that would otherwise go into digestion. It is believed that this diverted energy contributes to a sensation of vigor by being available for other essential functions.

Consistent Energy Release: Throughout the day, whole, plant-based foods like fruits and vegetables offer a consistent release of energy. By avoiding processed and sugary foods, blood sugar levels can be stabilized and energy dumps can be avoided.

Improved Physical Performance: A few people who follow the Mucusless Diet claim to have experienced increases in their stamina and physical performance. Plant-based diets are rich in nutrients, which may improve general health and fitness.

Many people who follow the Mucusless Diet report feeling more energized, alert, and focused than they did before they started following the diet. Individual responses to dietary changes can vary.

Weight Management and Body Composition

Balancing the Scales Through Nutrient-Dense Choices

A popular health objective is to acquire and maintain a healthy body composition, and the Mucusless Diet is frequently explored by persons who are interested in achieving and maintaining a healthy body composition. It is consistent with the principles linked with weight management that the diet emphasizes plant-based foods that are rich in nutrients.

Plant-Based Whole Foods: Since plant-based foods are typically higher in fiber and lower in calories, they are emphasized in the Mucusless

Diet. This strategy can help with weight management because it lowers total caloric intake and encourages feelings of fullness.

Avoiding Processed Foods: The Mucusless Diet restricts processed foods, which are frequently heavy in harmful fats and added sugars. By limiting the intake of calorie-dense, nutrient-poor alternatives, this restriction may help with weight management.

Enhanced Sensitivity to Cues of Hungry and Fullness: Those who adhere to the Mucusless Diet may have an elevated sense of hunger and fullness due to its emphasis on whole foods and mindful eating. By encouraging attentive eating, overeating can be avoided and good eating habits can be supported.

Although maintaining a healthy weight involves a complicated interaction of factors such as genetics, physical activity, and lifestyle choices, the Mucusless Diet provides a dietary framework that is in line with these fundamental concepts.

Enhancing Mental Clarity and Emotional Well-being

Nourishing the Mind and Spirit Through Dietary Choices

The Mucusless Diet is not just concerned with the physical components of health; it also highlights the connection between dietary choices and mental clarity, emotional well-being, and general spiritual health.

Those who follow the Mucus-Free Diet frequently report seeing a reduction in the amount of brain fog they experience as well as an increase in their mental clarity. When it comes to improving cognitive function, it is considered that avoiding certain meals that cause mucus formation can be beneficial.

Emotional equilibrium: the connection between one's nutrition and mood is a complicated and multi-faceted web of relationships. Nevertheless, some people follow the Mucusless Diet and claim to have experienced an improvement in their mental well-being. They attribute this improvement to the comprehensive character of the nutritional approach.

Spiritual Connection: The Mucusless Diet is not just a physical discipline for some people, but it also has a spiritual connection for others. The holistic approach to the diet, which helps to develop a sense of oneness and balance, is founded on the notion that the body, mind, and spirit are all interconnected with one another.

A significant number of individuals who adhere to the Mucusless Diet report feeling a sense of mental clarity, emotional equilibrium, and spiritual connectedness. This is even though the subjective nature of mental and emotional experiences makes it difficult to quantify these benefits using scientific methods.

CHAPTER 6: INTEGRATING MUCUSLESS DIET INTO LIFESTYLE

The adoption of the Mucusless Diet entails more than just making decisions about what to eat; it also involves making significant changes to one's lifestyle. The purpose of this part is to discuss how to incorporate the Mucusless Diet into various facets of your life. Topics that are covered include physical activity, mindfulness, stress management, social elements, dining out, and even navigating food choices while traveling.

Mucusless Diet and Physical Activity

- ## Synergy for Holistic Wellness

Participating in physical activity is an essential element of leading a healthy lifestyle, and combining it with the Mucusless Diet has the potential to magnify the advantages of both factors. To make the Mucusless Diet compatible with your exercise regimen, here is how to do it:

- Selecting Energizing Foods: During physical activity, choose foods that offer long-lasting energy without triggering upset stomachs. Fruits are a great pre-workout food, especially those high in carbs.

- Keep Yourself Hydrated: Staying well hydrated is crucial for the Mucusless Diet and physical activity. During exercise, water helps with temperature regulation, nutrient transfer, and digestion.

- Post-Workout Recovery: Consume foods high in nutrients to refuel your body after working out. Consume fruits, vegetables, and plant-based proteins to aid in the healing of your muscles and your general health.

- Exercises that are in tune with your body and mind should be done with mindfulness. Whether it's weight training, yoga, or running, pick exercises that suit your interests and energy levels.

You may develop a synergistic approach to well-being by combining the concepts of the Mucusless Diet with an active lifestyle. This will promote the natural detoxification processes that occur within your body and enhance your overall vitality.

Mindfulness and Stress Management

- ## **Balancing the Mind for Optimal Health**

When it comes to the comprehensive well-being that the Mucusless Diet seeks to promote, mindfulness and stress management are two of the most important factors. It is possible to contribute to a harmonious interaction between the mind and the body by incorporating these practices into your lifestyle:

- Savoring every bite, focusing on flavors, and being present throughout meals are all examples of mindful eating. This encourages a healthy digestive system in addition to improving the eating experience.

- Stress Reduction Methods: Include stress-reduction methods in your daily routine, like mindful walks, deep breathing exercises, and meditation. The Mucusless Diet's emphasis on fostering an interior environment that promotes healing is enhanced by these behaviors.

- Understanding the connection between physical and mental health is essential to holistic wellness. In line with the tenets of the Mucusless Diet, you can promote a comprehensive feeling of wellness by controlling stress and encouraging mindfulness in daily living.

The transforming effects of the Mucusless Diet are strengthened by a lifestyle that is balanced and aware, which further contributes to the development of a state of internal harmony and well-being.

Social Aspects and Dining Out

- **Navigating Social Situations with Ease**

Maintaining a mucus-free diet does not require one to give up the pleasure of dining out or the social ties that come with it. When going out to eat, here is how to handle social situations and make decisions based on accurate information:

- It's All About Communication: Inform friends and family about your dietary choices and limitations in plain language. By expressing your dedication to the Mucusless Diet, you can win over people to your way of thinking.

- Make Sensible Restaurant Selections: When dining out, pick establishments that provide a wide selection of fresh, plant-based dishes. Finding meals that fit the Mucusless Diet is now easier because so many restaurants now accommodate a wide range of dietary requirements.

- Change Menu Options: Feel free to make any changes to your order. For dietary requirements, the majority of eateries are flexible and willing to make modifications. Ask for a dish that is solely composed of vegetables and excludes specific ingredients.

- Be Ready: Think about bringing a food that fits the Mucusless Diet to offer when you attend social events. This guarantees that you have a healthy choice and shares with others the mouthwatering benefits of the Mucusless Diet.

Maintaining the Mucusless Diet's durability requires striking a balance between social interactions and nutritional choices. You can have pleasure in social interactions while adhering to your health objectives if you approach them with adaptability and honest communication.

Traveling on a Mucusless Diet

- **Exploring the World While Nourishing the Body**

When traveling, you may frequently encounter a variety of cuisines and nutritional options; but, if you make the necessary preparations, you will be able to adhere to the Mucusless Diet while discovering new places:

Investigate Local Food: Find options that are Mucusless and Diet-friendly by researching the local cuisine before your trip. This enables you to choose wisely and find delicious new recipes that fit your dietary requirements.

Bring Snacks: Bring snacks that are suitable for the Mucusless Diet during the trip. Keeping wholesome snacks on hand guarantees that you will have healthful options when traveling or in places where there may not be enough wholesome meals.

Share Dietary Needs: Be sure to share your dietary requirements with staff members when dining at restaurants or lodging. Special requests can be accommodated by many locations, ensuring that your meals follow the guidelines of the Mucusless Diet.

Explore Local Markets: Go to your local market to find fresh produce, fruits, and other ingredients that are suitable for the Mucusless Diet. This immerses you in the local cuisine culture while also enabling you to stick to your diet.

It is possible to journey around the world while adhering to the principles of the Mucusless Diet if you approach travel with a spirit of excitement and a feeling of preparation.

CHAPTER 7: COMMON MISCONCEPTIONS AND FAQS

When beginning a journey with the Mucusless Diet, it is possible that several questions and, at times, misconceptions will arise. In this area, we will attempt to dispel some of the most widespread misconceptions about the Mucusless Diet, as well as provide detailed responses to some of the most often-asked questions.

Addressing Myths and Misunderstandings

- **Separating Fact from Fiction**

Due to its unusual dietary recommendations and guiding ideas, the Mucusless Diet has given rise to several misconceptions. It is imperative to tackle these myths in order to promote a more precise comprehension of the diet:

- Myth: The Body Is Capable of Excluding All Mucus: A prevalent misperception is that adhering to the Mucusless Diet results in a body devoid of mucus entirely. Mucus production is a normal and necessary function of the human body, especially in the digestive and respiratory systems. By

93

avoiding particular foods, the diet aims to lessen excessive mucus production.

- Myth: All Grains Are Bad: The Mucusless Diet does not completely ban all grains, but it does advise restricting certain of them. When consumed in moderation, whole grains like quinoa and brown rice are seen as appropriate. The focus is on staying away from processed and refined grains.

- Myth: The Diet Is Insufficient in Protein: It is a common misperception that a plant-based diet—like the Mucusless Diet—is insufficient in protein. As it happens, plant-based protein-rich meals, legumes, nuts, and seeds are all part of a well-planned Mucusless Diet.

Individual demands for protein can differ, though.

- Myth: There Is No One-Size-Fits-All Method: A common misconception about the Mucusless Diet is that it's a strict, one-size-fits-all method. In actuality, the diet is flexible and adaptable to personal tastes, health objectives, and cultural factors. It's critical to modify the diet to meet each person's needs.

- Myth: You Must Complete Detoxification Quickly: Some may think that part of the Mucusless Diet is fast detoxification, which is marked by strong symptoms. Although detox symptoms are possible, the diet recommends a gradual shift to reduce discomfort and promote long-term adherence.

By addressing these fallacies, people can get rid of preconceptions and approach the Mucusless Diet with a clearer knowledge of its guiding principles and objectives.

Frequently Asked Questions about the Mucusless Diet

- **Providing Clarity on Common Queries**

Questions about the Mucusless Diet may come up when people learn more about it. Answering common queries demystifies the diet and gives prospective or current adherents of its principles clarity:

Q1: Can I follow the Mucusless Diet and still obtain adequate nutrients?

A1: Yes, if followed correctly, the Mucusless Diet can supply enough amount of nutrients. To provide a wide range of vital vitamins, minerals, and other nutrients, it emphasizes a variety of fruits, vegetables, grains, nuts, and seeds.

Q2: Is the Mucusless Diet appropriate for people who need a lot of energy, like athletes?

A2: Athletes or those with high energy requirements might modify the Mucusless Diet to suit their needs. It can support physical activity and energy demands by including whole grains, plant-based protein sources, and calorie-dense fruits.

Q3: How can I go from my current diet to the Mucusless Diet without going through detoxification?

A3: It is advised to transfer gradually to reduce detox symptoms. Increase the number of items that fit the Mucusless Diet progressively while lowering the number of meals that cause mucus. Getting enough sleep and drinking plenty of water might also help to facilitate a seamless shift.

Q4: Can children follow the Mucusless Diet?

A4: With the right adjustments, children can follow the Mucusless Diet and guarantee they get the nutrients they need for healthy growth and development. It is best to speak with a pediatrician or nutritionist to customize a diet for a child's unique requirements.

Q5: Will the Mucusless Diet be beneficial for treating particular medical concerns like skin diseases or allergies?

A5: Although anecdotal data indicates that people have seen improvements in a variety of health concerns, there is a dearth of scientific studies on the precise advantages of the mucusless diet. It's critical to view the diet as a whole lifestyle decision and seek the guidance of medical professionals for individualized recommendations.

Clarifying Concerns and Debunking Myths

- ## Promoting Informed Decision-Making

Beyond particular queries, people could have worries or run against enduring misconceptions. It is crucial to address these issues to promote well-informed decision-making:

Concern: Lack of Diversity in Food Choices

Clarification: Although there is a large selection of fruits, vegetables, cereals, nuts, and seeds to pick from, the Mucusless Diet may initially appear to be limited. People can enjoy a varied and fulfilling selection of meals that are suitable for the Mucusless Diet with a little imagination and inquiry.

Concern: Social Isolation and Limited Dining Options

Clarification: Embracing the Mucusless Diet does not imply social distancing. It might be beneficial to have an open dialogue regarding food choices with loved ones to foster understanding and support. The availability of plant-based menu items at many restaurants has made it feasible to follow the guidelines of the Mucusless Diet when eating out.

Concern: Lack of Scientific Evidence

Clarification: Concerns regarding the scant scientific data in favor of the Mucusless Diet may be voiced by some people. Although there isn't much study on this particular dietary strategy, the diet is in line with the ideas of plant-based nutrition, which has been connected to several health advantages. It is imperative that one approach the Mucusless Diet with an open mind and the readiness to modify in light of personal experience.

Concern: Perceived Complexity and Rule Adherence

Clarification: The Mucusless Diet's recommendations for foods that cause mucus may at first seem complicated. People can, however, approach it flexibly and modify it to fit their needs and interests. The diet promotes a gradual shift, enabling people to discover a balance that suits them.

CHAPTER 8: LONG-TERM MAINTENANCE AND CONTINUED HEALING

Beginning the journey of the Mucusless Diet is not just a short-term commitment; rather, it is a transformation in lifestyle that is intended to create long-term well-being. In this section, an examination of the evolving science and research on the Mucusless Diet is presented, as well as strategies for monitoring and adjusting the Mucusless Diet over time, preventing relapses and setbacks, integrating Mucusless principles for optimal wellness throughout one's entire life, and integrating Mucusless principles.

Monitoring and Adjusting Your Mucusless Diet

- ## Adapting to Changing Needs

It's critical to keep an eye on how your body is responding to the Mucusless Diet and to adapt as needed. The following are important factors for ongoing maintenance:

Frequent Self-Reflection: Make time to regularly reflect on your general well-being, energy levels, and health. Examine how your body reacts to various foods and record any changes in your overall health.

Pay Attention to Your Body: Pay attention to your body's cues. Think about making changes to your Mucusless Diet if you notice any changes in your energy levels, digestion, or other health indicators.

Include Variety: To guarantee a wide range of nutrients, keep your mucusless diet varied. To keep your diet varied and engaging, try different fruits, vegetables, grains, nuts, and seeds.

Speak with Experts: To make sure that your food choices support your health objectives, periodically consult with nutritionists or healthcare professionals. They can offer tailored advice depending on your particular requirements and state of health.

Adjusting your Mucusless Diet over time offers flexibility and ensures that the diet continues to be a part of your lifestyle that is both sustainable and pleasurable.

Preventing Relapses and Setbacks

- **Building Resilience for Consistency**

There is a possibility of experiencing occasional relapses or setbacks, even though the Mucusless Diet is beneficial to long-term health. The following is a guide on avoiding and navigating them:

- Develop Mindfulness: Remind yourself of the effects of the food you choose on your health. You can prevent impulsive decisions that could cause relapses by practicing mindfulness.

- Acquire Knowledge from Failures: If you encounter a setback, see it as a chance to grow. Determine the causes of the gap and think about future strategies to deal with them. Make the most of setbacks as opportunities for development.

- Create a Support Network: Assemble a network of people who appreciate and comprehend your eating decisions. Having a support system of friends, family, or other Mucusless Diet adherents can help try times.

- Achievable and reasonable goals should be set for your Mucusless Diet. Setting unrealistic expectations can make you feel frustrated and make failure more likely.

Acknowledge minor triumphs and make strides toward long-term objectives.

Long-term success with the Mucusless Diet can be achieved through the cultivation of resilience and the adoption of a proactive mindset. This will allow you to overcome obstacles and continue to adhere to the diet.

Integrating Mucusless Principles for Lifelong Wellness

Beyond Diet: A Comprehensive Strategy for Well-Being.

The Mucusless Diet is a comprehensive approach to health that goes beyond just what you eat. Think about these guidelines for enduring well-being:

Holistic Self-Care: Take a holistic approach to taking care of yourself by including activities that support your mental, emotional, and physical health. This could involve thoughtful activities, frequent exercise, stress reduction methods, and restful sleep.

Mind-Body Connection: Develop an understanding of how the mind and body are related. Recognize the impact your ideas and feelings can have on your physical well-being. Techniques like mindfulness and meditation can strengthen this bond.

Lifelong Learning: Continue your education throughout your life to stay educated about wellness and health. Attend seminars, look at new studies, and keep an open mind about how viewpoints on nutrition and well-being are changing.

Pay Attention to Your Body's Signals: Your body gives you insightful information. Pay attention to cues including appetite, fullness, and energy levels. As your body's needs change over time, make adjustments to your food and way of living.

An all-encompassing approach to well-being that incorporates Mucusless principles lays the groundwork for long-term health and vigor.

The Evolving Science and Research on Mucusless Diet

- **Staying Informed in a Dynamic Landscape**

A growing interest in plant-based nutrition and holistic health is driving scientific investigation into dietary alternatives such as the Mucusless Diet. Keep up with the latest developments in science and research:

Scientific Research: Although there isn't much data on the Mucusless Diet specifically, there is plenty to learn about plant-based nutrition in general and how it affects health. The advantages of eating a diet high in fruits,

115

vegetables, and whole grains have been shown in several studies.

Examine Emerging Findings: Pay attention to any new information regarding the Mucusless Diet. As scientific knowledge advances, further investigations may shed light on the advantages and disadvantages of this nutritional strategy.

Critical Evaluation: Have a critical attitude when reading scientific publications. Analyze research papers' general quality, sample sizes, and methodology. Examine the results from the perspective of the larger area of nutrition.

Seek Advice from Experts: If in doubt, seek advice from registered dietitians or other medical specialists with experience in plant-based nutrition. They can assist you in making decisions by providing advice based on the most recent scientific data.

Keeping up to date with scientific developments enables you to make decisions based on facts and modify your Mucusless Diet strategy in response to emerging information.

CONCLUSION

As we come to the end of this investigation into the Mucusless Diet Healing System, it is appropriate to contemplate the fundamentals, support ongoing healing, and think about the potential of this dietary approach in the context of holistic health and wellness.

Recapitulation of Mucusless Diet Principles

Essentials for Well-Being and Energy

The early 20th-century origins of the Mucusless Diet have drawn attention to its focus on removing items that cause mucus to enhance health and vitality. Let's review the fundamental ideas that underpin this eating strategy:

Steer Clear of Foods That Form Mucus: The main tenet of the mucusless diet is avoiding items that are thought to increase mucus formation. Dairy, processed foods, and specific cereals fall within this category.

Focus on Entire, Plant-Based Foods: Fruits, vegetables, nuts, seeds, and grains are among the whole, plant-based foods that are encouraged to be consumed as part of this diet. These foods are thought to assist the body's natural healing processes since they are high in vital nutrients.

Appropriate Food Combining: To maximize digestion, the Mucusless Diet promotes appropriate food combining. This includes recommendations like consuming fruits on an empty stomach and steering clear of pairing proteins with carbohydrates.

Gradual Transition: The Mucusless Diet advocates for a gradual transition since it understands the difficulties associated with sudden dietary changes. This strategy seeks to lessen detox symptoms and assist people in adjusting to a new diet.

Beyond food recommendations, the Mucusless Diet encourages a holistic perspective on health that takes into account the connections between mental, emotional, and physical well-being.

Restating these guidelines serves as a reminder of the Mucusless Diet's holistic approach—a way of life that goes beyond the plate to include a variety of facets of health.

Encouragement and Motivation for Continued Healing

Accepting the Path to Well-Being

Making a big nutritional change, like switching to the Mucusless Diet, is a journey that takes time, patience, and introspection. Here's some inspiration for ongoing healing and support for individuals who are on this path:

Celebrate Your Progress: Let yourself know how far you've come on the Mucusless Diet. Honoring your accomplishments strengthens your resolve to take care of your body, whether it's through better digestion, more energy, or a closer relationship with it.

Recognize that the Mucusless Diet is not a set of inflexible guidelines; instead, adapt and learn. It's a framework that you may modify to fit your unique requirements and changing perspective on health. Acquire knowledge from your encounters, adapt, and maintain an open mind to further develop.

Mindful Living: Think beyond the box when it comes to the Mucusless Diet. Incorporate habits that feed your mind and spirit to embrace a mindful life. This could involve engaging in joyful and fulfilling activities, frequent exercise, and meditation.

Community and Support: Make connections with people who have similar health goals to your own. Creating a community of support for yourself on your healing journey offers inspiration, a sense of togetherness, and shared experiences.

Self-compassion: Treat oneself with kindness. As healing is a process, obstacles are normal to face along the route. Remember that every day is an opportunity to make decisions that support your well-being and cultivate self-compassion.

Sustaining healing with the Mucusless Diet is a journey of self-discovery and well-being rather than a destination. With passion and a dedication to taking care of your body, mind, and soul, embrace the trip.

The Future of Mucusless Diet and Holistic Well-being

A   Changing   Environment   for   Health Consciousness

A number of things spring to mind when we think about the Mucusless Diet's future and its place in the field of holistic well-being:

Integration with Current Nutrition Science: The Mucusless Diet, which has its roots in theories from the early 20th century, can gain by being integrated with current nutrition science. An increasingly sophisticated understanding of the diet's effects on health can be attained through ongoing studies on plant-based diets, gut health, and holistic well-being.

Tailored Strategies: Holistic well-future beings acknowledge the significance of customized methods to health. The Mucusless Diet may be more relevant and successful if it is modified to account for the fact that people differ in their dietary requirements, tastes, and health situations.

Cultural Sensitivity: Cultural settings have a profound impact on holistic well-being. Although it offers broad guidelines, the Mucusless Diet can develop into a more culturally aware approach that takes into account different eating customs and tastes.

Collaboration with Healthcare Specialists: As interest in holistic health methods increases, people following the Mucusless Diet must work closely with healthcare professionals. It is possible to make sure that dietary decisions support personal health objectives by incorporating the knowledge of licensed dietitians, nutritionists, and medical specialists.

Holistic Wellness Platforms: The Mucusless Diet can potentially be shared through holistic wellness platforms in the digital age. Knowledge-sharing, support networks, and continuous learning can be facilitated by mobile applications, online communities, and educational materials.

The Mucusless Diet can work in harmony with new developments in holistic health in the future, adding to a more thorough knowledge of health that includes dietary decisions, awareness, and the interdependence of the body, mind, and spirit.